Somatic Exercises and

Integrating Mindful Movements and Practices for
Holistic Health

Eliora Penrose

Disclaimer

The information provided in this book, "Somatic Exercises and Wellness: Integrating Mindful Movements and Practices for Holistic Health," is for educational and informational purposes only. The content is not intended as medical or healthcare advice and should not be used for diagnosing or treating a health problem or disease. It is not a substitute for professional medical advice, diagnosis, or treatment.

Always seek the advice of your physician or other qualified health provider with any questions you may have regarding a medical condition. Never disregard professional medical advice or delay in seeking it because of something you have read in this book.

The author and publisher are not responsible for any specific health or allergy needs that may require medical supervision and are not liable for any damages or negative consequences from any treatment, action, application, or preparation, to any person reading or following the information in this book. References are provided for informational purposes only and do not constitute an endorsement of any sources.

Contents

Preface

Embracing the Dance of Body and Mind: The Pathway to Holistic Harmony

In the intricate tapestry of modern life, where the rhythm of our days often leads us away from the core of our being, the quest for a practice that reunites the body with the mind becomes not just essential but life-affirming. This book, " **Somatic Exercises and Wellness: Integrating Mindful Movements and Practices for Holistic Health** " is an invitation to embark on such a transformative journey. It is a journey that views movement not merely as physical activity but as a gateway to deeper self-awareness and comprehensive well-being.

This guide ventures beyond the traditional confines of physical fitness and weight management. It is not a tale of grueling workouts or restrictive diets. Instead, it is a narrative about attuning oneself to the nuanced languages of the body and mind. Our goal is to introduce you to practices that foster this connection, focusing on gentle, mindful movements that aid in achieving sustainable health goals, including weight loss, and more importantly, in nurturing overall wellness.

Blending principles from various somatic disciplines, mindfulness techniques, and nutritional wisdom, the book presents a well-rounded approach to health. It is designed to be inclusive, welcoming individuals of all ages and fitness levels. The practices and philosophies detailed in these pages are meant for daily integration, making wellness an organic and enjoyable part of your life's rhythm.

As you turn these pages, remember that the journey of somatic wellness transcends physical transformation. It is about cultivating a relationship with your body that is rooted in compassion, understanding, and respect. It is about seeking balance, not only physically but in all aspects of life.

With an open mind and heart, embark on this explorative journey. This book is your companion in discovering the harmonious blend of movement, mindfulness, and nourishment. Let it be the beginning of a path toward a more connected, vibrant, and fulfilling existence.

Welcome to a world where wellness is a dance of body and mind, a continuous, enriching experience. Your journey to holistic harmony begins here.

With warmth and encouragement,

Eliora Penrose

Introduction to Somatic Wellness

What is Somatic Wellness?

Somatic Wellness is an approach to health and fitness that emphasizes the deep connection between the mind and the body. Originating from the Greek word "soma," which means the living body, somatic practices focus on the body's internal experiences—such as movement, sensation, and perception—rather than just external appearances or performance metrics. This holistic approach integrates physical movement, mindfulness, and an awareness of the interconnectedness of mental and physical health.

The Core Principles of Somatic Wellness

1. **Body Awareness**: Recognizing and understanding the sensations, movements, and signals of the body.

2. **Mindfulness**: Cultivating a state of active, open attention to the present moment, which is integrated into movement practices.

3. **Holistic Health**: Viewing physical fitness not as an isolated activity but as part of a broader spectrum of well-being that includes mental, emotional, and spiritual health.

4. **Self-Regulation and Autonomy**: Encouraging individuals to take charge of their own health and wellness journey by listening to their body's unique needs and responses.

How Somatic Wellness Differs from Traditional Exercise

Unlike traditional exercise regimes that often prioritize external goals such as weight loss, muscle gain, or performance, Somatic Wellness focuses on the internal experience of movement. It is less about how exercises look and more about how they feel. This internal focus helps in developing a deeper connection with one's body, leading to more sustainable and meaningful health outcomes.

The Benefits of Somatic Wellness

- **Improved Mind-Body Connection**: Enhances the awareness and synchronization between mental and physical states.

- **Reduced Stress and Anxiety**: Mindfulness and body-centered practices are known to lower stress levels and promote mental clarity.

- **Increased Flexibility and Mobility**: Focuses on natural movements that improve the body's range of motion and reduce stiffness.

- **Sustainable Weight Management**: Encourages a healthy and balanced approach to weight loss that is sustainable in the long term.

Somatic Wellness and Sustainable Weight Loss

In the context of weight loss, Somatic Wellness offers a unique perspective. It advocates for a gradual, mindful approach to body transformation, emphasizing self-compassion and awareness over rapid, often unsustainable methods. This approach not only helps in achieving weight loss goals but also in maintaining them through a deeper understanding and respect for the body.

Conclusion

Somatic Wellness is more than just a fitness trend; it's a comprehensive approach to living that encourages individuals to harmoniously align their physical and mental well-being. By emphasizing internal awareness, mindfulness, and holistic health, it offers a path to sustainable wellness and a healthier, more balanced lifestyle.

The Philosophy Behind Integrating Mind, Body, and Spirit for Weight Loss

Understanding the Triad: Mind, Body, and Spirit

The integration of mind, body, and spirit forms the foundation of a holistic approach to weight loss. This philosophy recognizes that sustainable weight loss and overall well-being are not solely about physical changes but involve a comprehensive transformation that encompasses mental, emotional, and spiritual health.

Mind: The Power of Thoughts and Emotions

- **Mental Health and Weight Loss**: Our thoughts and emotions play a crucial role in our eating habits and physical health. Stress, anxiety, and negative self-perception can lead to unhealthy eating patterns.

- **Positive Mindset**: Cultivating a positive mindset, including self-acceptance and self-love, is essential for lasting weight loss. It involves changing how we think about food, our bodies, and the process of losing weight.

- **Mindfulness Practices**: Incorporating mindfulness can help in being present during meals, understanding hunger cues, and enjoying food more healthily.

Body: The Physical Aspect of Wellness

- **Physical Health and Weight Loss**: The body aspect involves regular physical activity, nutrition, and understanding the body's needs. It's about finding balance, not extreme measures.

- **Somatic Exercises**: These exercises encourage deeper body awareness and help in identifying tension and stress points, leading to more effective and enjoyable movement.

- **Nutritional Awareness**: Understanding how different foods affect the body and choosing a diet that supports physical health and weight loss goals.

Spirit: The Role of Inner Peace and Connection

- **Spiritual Wellness**: This encompasses a sense of connection to something greater than oneself and can be crucial for motivation and resilience in the weight loss journey.

- **Inner Peace**: Achieving inner peace through practices like meditation, yoga, or prayer can provide the strength and clarity needed for weight loss and maintenance.

- **Harmony and Balance**: Spirituality in the context of weight loss is about finding harmony and balance in life, aligning one's actions with deeper values and purposes.

Integrating Mind, Body, and Spirit

- **Holistic Approach**: This approach to weight loss is about creating harmony between the mind, body, and spirit. It's a journey of self-discovery and transformation that goes beyond the scale.

- **Sustainable Change**: By addressing all aspects of self, changes made are more likely to be sustainable. This method moves away from quick fixes to long-term lifestyle changes.

- **Empowerment and Self-Care**: The integration empowers individuals to take charge of their health in a compassionate and nurturing way, viewing weight loss as a form of self-care and self-respect.

Conclusion

The philosophy of integrating mind, body, and spirit for weight loss is a comprehensive, compassionate, and sustainable approach. It acknowledges the complexity of weight loss and promotes a more fulfilling and holistic path to health and wellness. By embracing this philosophy, individuals embark on a journey that not only transforms their body but also enriches their mind and nourishes their spirit.

Chapter 1: Understanding Somatic Wellness

The Concept of Somatic Exercises

Definition and Origins

"Somatic" exercises, derived from the Greek word "soma" meaning "living body," are a form of physical exercise focusing on the internal experience of movement and body awareness. This approach was developed with the understanding that the mind and body are interconnected and that physical movement can influence mental and emotional well-being.

Principles of Somatic Exercises

1. **Internal Focus**: Unlike traditional exercises that often emphasize external outcomes (like muscle gain or weight loss), somatic exercises prioritize the internal experience — how movements feel in the body.

2. **Mindfulness and Movement**: These exercises incorporate mindfulness, making practitioners aware of their bodily sensations and movements in real-time.

3. **Gentle and Holistic**: Somatic exercises are typically gentle, emphasizing smooth movements that integrate the whole body rather than isolating specific muscles.

4. **Self-Healing and Empowerment**: They empower individuals to explore and understand their bodies, often leading to self-healing and improved overall functioning.

Types of Somatic Exercises

- **Hanna Somatics**: Focuses on re-educating the body and mind in movement patterns, often used for pain relief and improved mobility.

- **Feldenkrais Method**: Enhances self-awareness through movement and aims to improve movement efficiency and body function.

- **Alexander Technique**: Teaches better posture and movement to reduce muscle tension and improve ease and efficiency of movement.

- **Body-Mind Centering**: A holistic approach that combines movement, voice, and mind to explore body systems, patterns, and dynamics.

How Somatic Exercises Work

- **Neuromuscular Movement**: These exercises involve slow, conscious movements that help retrain the neuromuscular system, enhancing body awareness and altering habitual movement patterns.

- **Release and Relaxation**: They often lead to the release of chronic muscular tension and promote relaxation and stress reduction.

- **Body Awareness**: Practitioners become more attuned to their body's needs, capabilities, and signals, leading to better overall body understanding and care.

Benefits of Somatic Exercises

1. **Improved Flexibility and Mobility**: Enhances the body's natural range of motion and reduces stiffness.

2. **Stress Reduction**: The mindful nature of somatic exercises helps in lowering stress and anxiety levels.

3. **Pain Management**: Effective in addressing chronic pain issues by altering habitual movement patterns that contribute to pain.

4. **Enhanced Body-Mind Connection**: Strengthens the connection between physical movement and mental states, leading to greater harmony and balance.

5. **Improved Posture and Balance**: Regular practice can lead to improved posture and balance, reducing the risk of falls and injuries.

Conclusion

Somatic exercises represent a profound shift from conventional exercise philosophy, focusing on the internal experience and the holistic integration of mind and body. By practicing these exercises, individuals can achieve a heightened sense of body awareness, improved physical health, and a deeper connection between their physical movements and emotional states. This approach is especially beneficial for those seeking a gentle yet effective pathway to physical wellness and mental clarity.

The Role of Mindfulness in Physical Health

Understanding Mindfulness

Mindfulness is a mental practice that involves maintaining a moment-by-moment awareness of our thoughts, feelings, bodily sensations, and the surrounding environment in a non-judgmental way. It often involves techniques such as meditation, deep breathing, and focusing on the present moment.

The Mind-Body Connection

- **Integrating Mind and Body**: Mindfulness strengthens the connection between the mind and the body. Being mindful about bodily states brings a deeper awareness of the physical self.

- **Stress Reduction**: Mindfulness is known to reduce stress, which can have a significant positive impact on physical health. Stress is a contributing factor to many chronic diseases, and its reduction can lead to better overall health.

Mindfulness in Health Behaviors

- **Conscious Eating**: Mindfulness encourages conscious eating, which can lead to healthier food choices and improved digestion.

- **Exercise and Mindfulness**: When exercise is performed mindfully, it can increase the effectiveness of the workout, reduce the risk of injury, and enhance enjoyment.

Impact on Chronic Conditions

- **Pain Management**: Mindfulness meditation has been shown to reduce pain sensations in the body and can be an effective tool in managing chronic pain.

- **Chronic Disease Management**: Mindfulness can help in managing chronic diseases like hypertension, heart disease, and diabetes by improving lifestyle choices and reducing stress-related impacts on the body.

Psychological Well-being and Physical Health

- **Reduced Anxiety and Depression**: Mindfulness practices can help reduce symptoms of anxiety and depression, which in turn can have a positive effect on physical health.

- **Improved Sleep**: Mindfulness techniques can contribute to better sleep quality, which is crucial for physical health and recovery.

Mindfulness and Immunity

- **Boosting Immune System**: Regular mindfulness practice has been linked to improved immune function, helping the body to fight off illness more effectively.

Enhancing Self-Awareness

- **Body Awareness**: Being mindful increases body awareness, helping individuals to recognize signs of physical discomfort or illness early, leading to prompt care and treatment.

- **Emotional Regulation**: It aids in recognizing and managing emotions, which can have a direct impact on physical health, such as reducing the incidence of stress-related disorders.

Conclusion

The role of mindfulness in physical health is multifaceted, impacting everything from stress reduction to chronic disease management. By fostering a deep connection between mind and body, mindfulness practices can lead to a healthier, more balanced life. This approach is not only preventative but also enhances the quality of life by improving physical health through a better understanding and management of emotional and psychological states.

Sustainable Weight Loss: A Holistic Approach
Defining Sustainable Weight Loss

Sustainable weight loss is an approach that focuses on long-term success rather than quick fixes. It involves making gradual lifestyle changes that can be maintained over time, rather than temporary diets or extreme exercise regimens. This holistic method considers the physical, mental, and emotional aspects of weight loss.

Physical Aspects of Sustainable Weight Loss

- **Balanced Diet**: Instead of restrictive diets, a balanced diet rich in nutrients supports long-term health and weight management.

- **Regular, Enjoyable Exercise**: Incorporating physical activities that are enjoyable and suitable for one's fitness level ensures consistency and sustainability.

- **Rest and Recovery**: Adequate sleep and rest are crucial for the body's metabolic processes and for maintaining energy levels.

Mental and Emotional Dimensions

- **Mindset Shift**: Changing one's mindset about weight loss from a short-term goal to a long-term health journey is essential.

- **Self-Compassion**: Practicing self-compassion and understanding that progress is not linear helps maintain motivation and reduces the likelihood of giving up.

- **Emotional Well-being**: Addressing emotional factors that contribute to weight gain, such as stress eating, through mindfulness and other stress-reduction techniques.

The Role of Mindfulness

- **Mindful Eating**: Being mindful while eating helps in recognizing true hunger cues, enjoying meals more, and avoiding overeating.

- **Awareness of Body's Needs**: Mindfulness promotes a better understanding of the body's needs, helping in making healthier choices.

Lifestyle and Environment

- **Healthy Environment**: Creating an environment that supports healthy eating and physical activity can significantly impact one's ability to maintain weight loss.

- **Community and Support**: Engaging with a community for support and accountability can be beneficial in staying on track.

Holistic Health Practices

- **Incorporating Holistic Practices**: Techniques such as yoga, meditation, and somatic exercises can enhance overall well-being and aid in weight management.

- **Alternative Therapies**: Exploring alternative therapies like acupuncture or aromatherapy can complement traditional weight loss methods and address other health concerns.

Education and Knowledge

- **Understanding Nutrition and Exercise**: Educating oneself about nutrition and exercise can empower one to make informed decisions.

- **Awareness of Body Mechanics**: Learning about body mechanics and how different exercises impact the body aids in choosing the most effective and safe activities.

Conclusion

Sustainable weight loss is a holistic approach that goes beyond mere calorie counting or intense workouts. It encompasses a balanced diet, regular physical activity, mental and emotional well-being, and a supportive environment. By focusing on long-term lifestyle changes and overall health, it offers a more achievable and healthy path to weight management.

Chapter 2: The Foundations of Somatic Movements

Principles of Somatic Exercises

Somatic exercises, rooted in the holistic understanding of the body, are designed to enhance physical well-being through mindful movement. These exercises are characterized by several key principles that distinguish them from traditional forms of exercise.

1. Body Awareness

- **Listening to the Body**: Somatic exercises emphasize tuning into the body's internal signals, understanding its needs and responses.

- **Sensory Feedback**: Practitioners are encouraged to pay close attention to the sensations that arise during movement, fostering a deeper connection with their physical self.

2. Mindfulness and Presence

- **Conscious Movement**: Each movement in somatic exercises is performed with full awareness and attention, keeping the mind present and engaged.

- **Mental Clarity**: This mindfulness aspect helps in achieving mental clarity and focus, reducing stress and enhancing the overall quality of the exercise.

3. Gentle and Controlled Movements

- **Non-Forceful Approach**: Somatic exercises involve gentle movements, avoiding any form of strain or force. They are low-impact and accessible to people of all ages and fitness levels.

- **Control and Precision**: Movements are executed with control and precision, prioritizing the quality of movement over quantity.

4. Integration of Mind and Body

- **Holistic Approach**: These exercises view the body and mind as an integrated unit, with each exercise designed to improve both physical and mental well-being.

- **Emotional Release**: As the body releases physical tension, there is often a corresponding release of emotional stress, fostering a sense of holistic healing.

5. Re-education of Movement

- **Correcting Patterns**: Somatic exercises help in re-educating the body to move in more efficient and healthier ways, correcting poor habitual movement patterns that may lead to pain or injury.

- **Neuromuscular Rebalancing**: By retraining the neuromuscular system, these exercises improve coordination, balance, and overall body function.

6. Self-Regulation and Autonomy

- **Empowering Individuals**: Practitioners are encouraged to explore movements independently, giving them autonomy over their practice and fostering self-regulation.

- **Adaptability**: Exercises can be adapted to meet individual needs, making them highly personalized and effective.

7. Breathing and Relaxation

- **Breath Integration**: Somatic exercises often incorporate intentional breathing, which aids in relaxation and enhances the effectiveness of movements.

- **Stress Reduction**: Focusing on breath helps in reducing stress and anxiety, further promoting a sense of calm and relaxation in the body.

8. Functional Movement

- **Everyday Movements**: The focus is on movements that are functional and can be translated into daily activities, improving the overall quality of life.

- **Efficiency and Ease**: These exercises aim to make everyday movements more efficient and effortless, reducing the risk of injury and increasing physical capability.

Conclusion

The principles of somatic exercises create a unique and effective approach to physical wellness. By emphasizing body awareness, mindfulness, gentle movement, and the integration of mind and body, these exercises offer a path to improved physical health, mental clarity, and emotional balance. This holistic approach not only enhances physical fitness but also contributes to overall life quality.

How Somatic Movements Differ from Traditional Exercises

Somatic movements and traditional exercises represent different philosophies and approaches towards physical health and fitness. Understanding these differences is crucial for appreciating the unique benefits of somatic practices.

1. Focus on Internal Experience vs. External Outcomes

- **Somatic Movements**: Prioritize the internal experience of movement — how the body feels and responds during the exercise.

- **Traditional Exercises**: Often focus on external outcomes like muscle gain, weight loss, or improved athletic performance.

2. Mindfulness and Body Awareness

- **Somatic Movements**: Involve a high degree of mindfulness, encouraging practitioners to be fully present and attentive to the sensations in their bodies.

- **Traditional Exercises**: May not emphasize mindfulness or the mental aspect of exercise, focusing more on physical exertion and achievement.

3. Gentle and Holistic Approach

- **Somatic Movements**: Typically gentle, designed to work with the body's natural rhythms and capacities, often suitable for all ages and fitness levels.

- **Traditional Exercises**: Can be more intense and rigorous, sometimes focusing on pushing the body to its limits.

4. Quality of Movement Over Quantity

- **Somatic Movements**: Emphasize the quality of movement, with a focus on how movements are performed rather than how many repetitions are completed.

- **Traditional Exercises**: Often emphasize the quantity of exercise, such as the number of repetitions, sets, or duration of the workout.

5. Individualized and Adaptive

- **Somatic Movements**: Highly adaptable to individual needs, focusing on personal comfort and the unique responses of one's body.

- **Traditional Exercises**: May follow a more one-size-fits-all approach, with standardized routines that don't always account for individual differences.

6. Integration of Mind, Body, and Emotion

- **Somatic Movements**: Aim to integrate the mind, body, and emotions, facilitating a holistic sense of well-being.

- **Traditional Exercises**: Typically focus primarily on physical aspects, with less emphasis on emotional or mental health.

7. Goal of Exercise

- **Somatic Movements**: Aim to increase body awareness, reduce stress, and improve overall bodily function.

- **Traditional Exercises**: Often aim to improve physical fitness, lose weight, or build muscle.

8. Approach to Pain and Discomfort

- **Somatic Movements**: Encourage gentle exploration of movements that can alleviate pain and discomfort.

- **Traditional Exercises**: Might push through pain as a part of the workout, adhering to the "no pain, no gain" mentality.

9. Long-term Perspective

- **Somatic Movements**: Focus on long-term health and sustainability, promoting practices that can be maintained throughout life.

- **Traditional Exercises**: Sometimes oriented towards short-term goals or gains, which might not always be sustainable.

Conclusion

Somatic movements offer a distinct approach to exercise that contrasts with traditional methods, prioritizing internal awareness, mindfulness, and the integration of the mind and body. This approach is often more about nurturing and understanding the body rather than pushing it to its limits, making it a valuable practice for long-term health and wellness.

The Mind-Body Connection in Somatic Wellness

Understanding the Mind-Body Connection

The mind-body connection in somatic wellness is based on the premise that the mind and body are not separate entities but are intricately connected and influence each other. This connection is central to somatic practices, which aim to harmonize this relationship for overall well-being.

Key Aspects of the Mind-Body Connection in Somatic Wellness

1. **Interplay Between Mental and Physical States**:

   - Emotions and thoughts can manifest physically in the body, often as tension or pain.

   - Conversely, physical states can influence mental and emotional well-being.

2. **Awareness and Perception**:

   - Somatic wellness encourages heightened awareness of bodily sensations and perceptions.

   - This increased awareness can lead to a deeper understanding of the body's needs and responses.

3. **Stress and Its Physical Manifestations**:

   - Stress can have significant physical implications, including muscle tension, headaches, and fatigue.

- Somatic practices often focus on relieving these physical symptoms of stress, thereby also alleviating mental stress.

4. **Movement and Emotional Release**:

   - Physical movements in somatic exercises can lead to the release of pent-up emotions.

   - This release is therapeutic, aiding in emotional processing and healing.

5. **Neuroplasticity and Habitual Patterns**:

   - Somatic exercises leverage neuroplasticity, the brain's ability to reorganize itself, to alter habitual movement and thought patterns that are detrimental.

   - By changing these patterns, individuals can improve their physical and mental health.

6. **Embodied Cognition**:

   - The concept that cognitive processes are deeply rooted in the body's interactions with the world.

   - Somatic wellness practices enhance this embodied cognition, leading to better decision-making and emotional regulation.

Benefits of the Mind-Body Connection in Somatic Wellness

- **Enhanced Overall Health**: By aligning the mind and body, individuals experience an overall improvement in health and well-being.

- **Improved Emotional Regulation**: Better body awareness leads to improved recognition and management of emotions.

- **Increased Resilience**: Strengthening the mind-body connection builds resilience against stress and adversity.

- **Greater Self-Awareness and Self-Care**: Individuals become more attuned to their needs and better equipped to care for themselves holistically.

Integrative Approach to Healing

- **Holistic Treatment**: Somatic wellness offers a holistic approach to treating various conditions, acknowledging that mental, emotional, and physical health are interconnected.

- **Preventative Care**: It serves as a form of preventative care, helping to maintain balance in the mind and body and ward off potential health issues.

Conclusion

The mind-body connection in somatic wellness is a fundamental aspect that drives its effectiveness. By fostering a deep, harmonious connection between the mind and body, somatic practices offer a powerful tool for holistic health, emotional healing, and personal growth. This approach underscores the importance of treating the individual as a whole, rather than focusing on isolated symptoms or aspects of well-being.

Chapter 3: Mindfulness Techniques for Wellness

Introduction to Mindfulness and Its Benefits

What is Mindfulness?

Mindfulness is a mental practice that involves maintaining a moment-to-moment awareness of our thoughts, feelings, bodily sensations, and the immediate environment in a non-judgmental and accepting manner. It is often cultivated through meditation but can also be practiced in daily activities.

Origins of Mindfulness

- **Historical Roots**: Mindfulness has its roots in ancient Eastern traditions, particularly Buddhism, but it has been adapted and secularized for use in Western health and psychology.

- **Modern Adaptation**: In recent decades, mindfulness has gained significant attention in the West for its therapeutic benefits and has been incorporated into various forms of therapy and wellness programs.

Core Principles of Mindfulness

1. **Present Moment Awareness**: Focusing on the here and now, rather than dwelling on the past or worrying about the future.

2. **Non-Judgmental Observation**: Observing thoughts and feelings without labeling them as good or bad.

3. **Acceptance**: Accepting things as they are without trying to change or resist them.

4. **Connection with Oneself**: Developing a deeper understanding and connection with oneself.

Benefits of Mindfulness

1. **Stress Reduction**: Mindfulness is known to reduce stress by promoting relaxation and emotional regulation.

2. **Improved Mental Health**: It can decrease symptoms of anxiety, depression, and improve overall psychological well-being.

3. **Enhanced Physical Health**: Benefits include lowered blood pressure, improved sleep, and enhanced immune function.

4. **Increased Focus and Concentration**: Regular mindfulness practice can improve attention, concentration, and decision-making skills.

5. **Emotional Regulation**: Helps in managing and understanding emotions more effectively.

6. **Better Pain Management**: Mindfulness can alter the perception of pain and aid in coping with chronic pain conditions.

7. **Improved Relationships**: By increasing empathy and compassion, mindfulness can enhance interpersonal relationships.

8. **Greater Resilience**: Builds resilience by fostering a more adaptable and positive response to challenges.

Mindfulness in Daily Life

- **Mindful Eating**: Paying full attention to the experience of eating and tasting food.

- **Mindful Walking**: Being fully present with each step and the sensations of walking.

- **Mindful Listening**: Actively listening and being present in conversations.

- **Mindfulness at Work**: Incorporating brief mindfulness exercises to reduce work-related stress and increase productivity.

Conclusion

Mindfulness is more than just a meditation practice; it's a way of living that fosters a deeper connection with oneself and the world. Its benefits extend across mental, emotional, and physical health, making it a powerful tool for enhancing overall well-being. By practicing mindfulness, individuals can cultivate a sense of peace, clarity, and balance in their lives.

Mindful Breathing and Meditation Practices

Introduction to Mindful Breathing

Mindful breathing is a fundamental aspect of mindfulness meditation. It involves focusing your attention on the breath, observing it as it flows in and out of the body, and using it as an anchor to the present moment.

Techniques of Mindful Breathing

1. **Basic Mindful Breathing**:

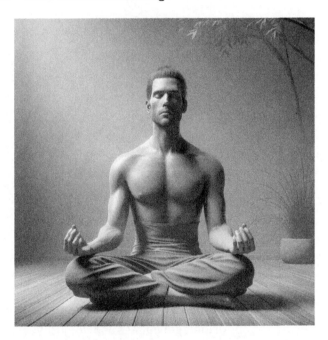

- Sit or lie down in a comfortable position.

- Close your eyes and bring your attention to your breath.

- Notice the sensation of air entering and leaving your nostrils, or the rise and fall of your chest or abdomen.

- If your mind wanders, gently bring your focus back to your breath.

2. **Deep Diaphragmatic Breathing**:

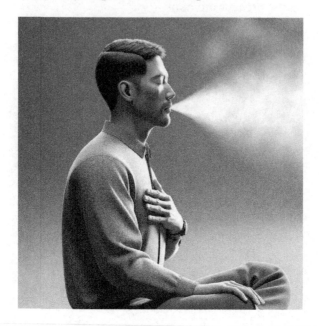

- Place one hand on your chest and the other on your abdomen.

- Breathe in deeply through your nose, ensuring your diaphragm inflates and not just your chest.

- Exhale slowly and deeply through the mouth.

- Focus on the movement of your diaphragm as you breathe.

3. **Counted Breathing**:

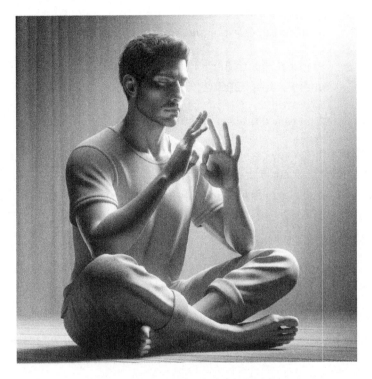

- Inhale while slowly counting to four.

- Hold your breath for a count of four.

- Exhale for a count of four.

- Pause for a count of four before the next breath.

Benefits of Mindful Breathing

- **Relaxation and Stress Reduction**: Slows down the heart rate and reduces stress hormone levels.

- **Improved Focus and Concentration**: Enhances the ability to concentrate and maintain attention.

- **Better Emotional Regulation**: Helps in managing anxiety, depression, and emotional outbursts.

- **Physical Health Benefits**: Can lower blood pressure and improve respiratory efficiency.

Introduction to Meditation Practices

Meditation, a key component of mindfulness, involves training the mind to focus and redirect thoughts. It can take many forms but generally includes techniques for relaxation, building internal energy, and developing compassion, love, patience, and forgiveness.

Common Meditation Practices

1. **Guided Meditation**:

   - Involves following a guided recording where an instructor leads you through a meditative practice.

   - Can include visualizations, body scans, or other mindfulness exercises.

2. **Mantra Meditation**:

   - Involves silently repeating a calming word, thought, or phrase to prevent distracting thoughts.

3. **Mindfulness Meditation**:

- Involves sitting silently and paying attention to thoughts, sounds, and sensations in a non-judgmental manner.

4. **Loving-kindness Meditation (Metta)**:

  - Involves mentally sending goodwill, kindness, and warmth towards others by silently repeating a series of mantras.

Integrating Meditation into Daily Life

- **Short, Regular Sessions**: Even 5-10 minutes of meditation daily can be beneficial.

- **Incorporating Mindfulness in Activities**: Practicing mindfulness during routine activities like eating, walking, or listening.

- **Creating a Dedicated Space**: Designate a quiet, comfortable space for meditation.

Conclusion

Mindful breathing and meditation practices are accessible tools that can significantly enhance mental and physical well-being. By regularly incorporating these practices into daily life, individuals can experience reduced stress, improved emotional well-being, enhanced concentration, and a deeper sense of overall calm and balance.

Applying Mindfulness in Everyday Life for Better Health

Introduction to Everyday Mindfulness

Mindfulness doesn't have to be limited to meditation sessions; it can be woven into the fabric of daily life. Practicing mindfulness in everyday activities can lead to significant improvements in overall health and well-being.

Mindful Eating

- **Eating with Attention**: Pay attention to the taste, texture, and aroma of your food. Chew slowly and savor each bite.

- **Listening to Hunger Cues**: Eat when you're hungry and stop when you're full, rather than eating out of boredom or emotion.

Mindful Walking

- **Awareness in Motion**: Focus on the sensation of your feet touching the ground, the rhythm of your steps, and your breathing.

- **Connection with the Environment**: Notice the sights, sounds, and smells around you as you walk.

Mindful Listening

- **Fully Engaging in Conversations**: Listen actively and attentively without planning your response while the other person is still talking.

- **Non-Judgmental Listening**: Listen without forming judgments or getting emotionally reactive to what is being said.

Mindfulness at Work

- **Mindful Breaks**: Take short breaks to breathe deeply or walk mindfully, especially during long periods of sitting or stressful tasks.

- **Single-Tasking**: Focus on one task at a time rather than multitasking, which can lead to increased stress and reduced productivity.

Mindful Relationships

- **Being Present with Others**: Give your full attention to others when interacting, without distractions from devices or your own thoughts.

- **Empathy and Understanding**: Practice understanding situations from others' perspectives, fostering deeper connections and empathy.

Mindful Leisure Activities

- **Engaging Fully in Activities**: Whether reading, gardening, or any hobby, immerse yourself fully in the activity without external distractions.

- **Appreciating the Moment**: Find joy in the process of the activity, not just the outcome.

Integrating Mindfulness into Daily Routines

- **Morning Routine**: Start the day with a few minutes of deep breathing or mindful stretching.

- **Mindful Commuting**: Use your commute as a time to decompress and transition between home and work life mindfully.

Mindfulness and Physical Health

- **Stress Management**: Regular mindfulness practice can reduce the physical effects of stress, such as high blood pressure and heart rate.

- **Improved Sleep**: Being mindful during the day can lead to better sleep quality at night.

Overcoming Challenges

- **Starting Small**: Begin with integrating mindfulness into one or two activities and gradually expand.

- **Dealing with Distractions**: Acknowledge distractions without judgment and gently bring your attention back to the present moment.

Conclusion

Incorporating mindfulness into everyday life can transform routine activities into opportunities for increased awareness, stress reduction, and enhanced well-being. By practicing mindfulness, you can cultivate a deeper connection with yourself and your environment, leading to better mental and physical health.

Chapter 4: Starting with Somatic Exercises

Basic Somatic Movements for Beginners

Somatic exercises are designed to reconnect the mind and body through gentle, mindful movements. They are particularly effective for beginners as they emphasize internal awareness over physical strain. Here are some basic somatic movements that beginners can easily incorporate into their routines.

1. The Cat-Cow Stretch

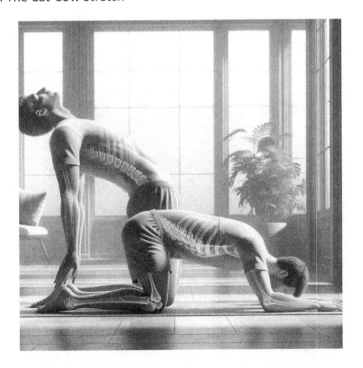

- **How to Perform:**

- Begin on your hands and knees in a tabletop position.

- As you inhale, arch your back, dropping your belly towards the floor (Cow position).

- As you exhale, round your spine towards the ceiling, tucking in your chin to your chest (Cat position).

- Continue to move slowly between these two positions, synchronizing your movement with your breath.

- **Benefits**: Improves spinal flexibility and awareness of spinal movement.

2. Pelvic Tilts

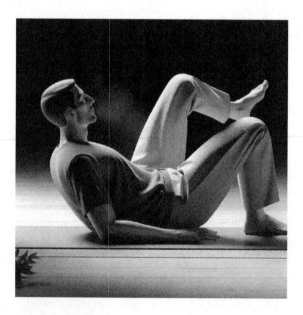

- **How to Perform**:

- Lie on your back with knees bent and feet flat on the floor.

- Inhale, allowing your pelvis to tilt forward, arching your lower back.

- Exhale, gently flattening your back against the floor.

- Repeat these tilts gently, focusing on the movement of the pelvis.

- **Benefits**: Enhances awareness of pelvic movements and relieves lower back tension.

3. Shoulder Rolls

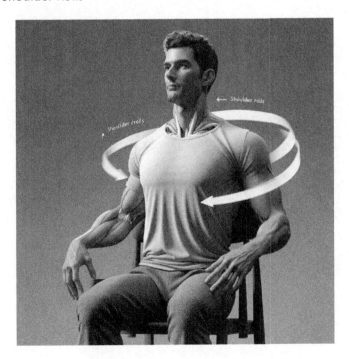

- **How to Perform**:

  - Sit or stand comfortably with your arms relaxed by your sides.

  - Slowly roll your shoulders up, then back, down, and forward in a smooth circular motion.

  - After a few repetitions, change direction and roll your shoulders forward, up, back, and down.

- **Benefits**: Releases tension in the shoulders and neck area.

4. Neck Turns

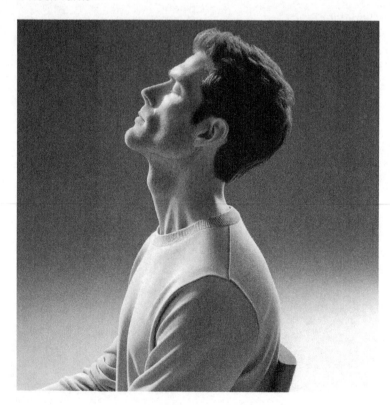

- **How to Perform**:

  - Sit up straight and slowly turn your head to the right as far as comfortable.

  - Hold for a moment, then slowly turn your head to the left.

  - Focus on the sensation of movement in your neck.

- **Benefits**: Increases neck mobility and awareness of neck tension.

5. Leg Extensions

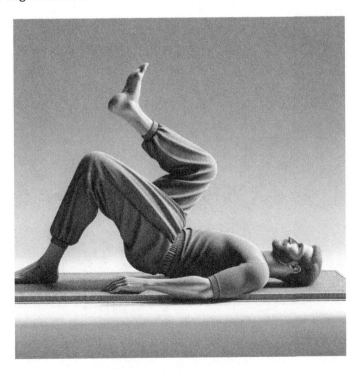

- **How to Perform**:

  - Lie on your back with both knees bent and feet flat on the floor.

  - Slowly straighten one leg, sliding your heel along the floor, then gently bring it back to the starting position.

  - Repeat with the other leg, maintaining a slow and mindful movement.

- **Benefits**: Gently stretches the legs and improves lower body awareness.

6. Arm Raises

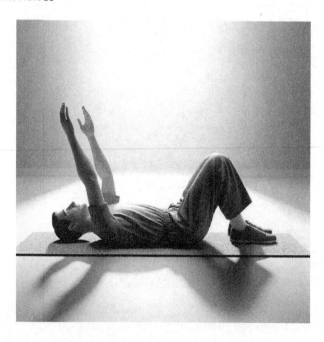

- **How to Perform**:

    - Lie on your back or sit comfortably.

    - Slowly raise your arms overhead, keeping them straight, and then lower them back down.

    - Coordinate the movement with your breath, raising arms on the inhale and lowering them on the exhale.

- **Benefits**: Enhances shoulder mobility and upper body awareness.

7. The Constructive Rest Position

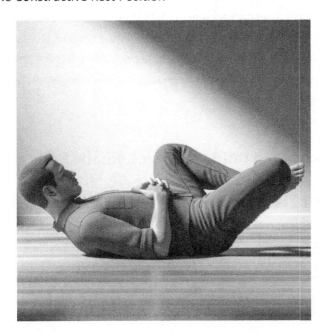

- **How to Perform**:

  - Lie on your back with knees bent and feet flat on the floor, hip-width apart.

  - Rest your hands on your abdomen or by your sides.

  - Stay in this position, breathing deeply and noticing the sensations in your body.

- **Benefits**: Encourages relaxation and body awareness.

Conclusion

These basic somatic movements are ideal for beginners to start developing body awareness and mindfulness. They can be performed daily and are particularly beneficial for those who spend long hours sitting or who experience chronic stress and tension. By practicing these exercises regularly, beginners can lay a strong foundation for improved mind-body connection and overall well-being.

Step-by-Step Guide to Basic Somatic Exercises for Beginners

Below are detailed instructions for each basic somatic exercise, ideal for beginners. These exercises focus on gentle movements and body awareness.

1. The Cat-Cow Stretch

Purpose: To increase spinal flexibility and awareness.

Steps:

1. Start on your hands and knees in a tabletop position, with your wrists directly under your shoulders and knees under hips.

2. Inhale, arch your back and tilt your pelvis up, dropping your belly towards the floor (Cow position).

3. Exhale, round your spine towards the ceiling and tuck your chin to your chest, pulling your belly in (Cat position).

4. Continue alternating between these positions for several breaths, moving smoothly with each inhale and exhale.

2. Pelvic Tilts

Purpose: To enhance pelvic mobility and relieve lower back tension.

Steps:

1. Lie on your back with your knees bent and feet flat on the floor, hip-width apart.

2. Inhale and gently arch your lower back, allowing a small space between your back and the floor.

3. Exhale and slowly flatten your back against the floor by tilting your pelvis upward.

4. Repeat this gentle rocking motion for several breaths, focusing on the movement of your pelvis.

3. Shoulder Rolls

Purpose: To release tension in the shoulders and neck.

Steps:

1.   Sit or stand comfortably with your spine straight.

2.   Inhale and lift your shoulders up towards your ears.

3.   Exhale and roll your shoulders back, drawing them down away from your ears.

4.   Continue this circular motion for several repetitions, then reverse the direction.

4. Neck Turns

Purpose: To increase neck mobility and reduce tension.

Steps:

1.   Sit comfortably with your spine erect.

2.   Slowly turn your head to the right, moving only as far as is comfortable. Pause and notice the stretch.

3.   Return to the center and repeat the movement to the left.

4.   Do several repetitions, maintaining a slow and mindful pace.

5. Leg Extensions

Purpose: To stretch and improve awareness of the lower body.

Steps:

1. Lie on your back with knees bent and feet flat on the floor.

2. Slowly extend one leg, sliding your heel along the floor until the leg is straight.

3. Pause and then slowly slide the heel back, returning to the starting position.

4. Repeat with the other leg, focusing on the movement and sensation in your legs.

6. Arm Raises

Purpose: To enhance shoulder mobility and upper body awareness.

Steps:

1. Lie on your back or sit with a straight spine.

2. Inhale and slowly raise your arms overhead, keeping them straight.

3. Exhale and gently lower them back to your sides.

4. Coordinate the movement with your breath, moving fluidly and attentively.

7. The Constructive Rest Position

Purpose: To promote relaxation and overall body awareness.

Steps:

1. Lie on your back with knees bent and feet flat on the floor, hip-width apart.

2.   Place your hands on your abdomen or by your sides.

3.   Breathe deeply, focusing on the rise and fall of your abdomen or chest.

4.   Stay in this position for several minutes, observing any sensations in your body.

Conclusion

These exercises should be performed slowly and with attention to the sensations in your body. They are not about reaching maximum stretch or strength but about connecting with and understanding your body. Regular practice can lead to improved mind-body awareness and overall well-being.

Customizing Your Somatic Routine for Weight Loss Goals

Understanding the Somatic Approach to Weight Loss

Somatic exercises for weight loss focus on body awareness and mindfulness, rather than intense calorie-burning activities. This approach can be highly effective for sustainable weight loss, as it encourages a deeper connection with the body and mindful lifestyle changes.

Tailoring Somatic Exercises to Your Needs

1.   **Identify Personal Goals**: Understand what you wish to achieve through your somatic practice. Is it just weight loss, or do you also want to improve flexibility, reduce stress, or alleviate pain?

2.   **Incorporate Cardiovascular Elements**: While somatic exercises are generally gentle, you can integrate light

cardiovascular activities like brisk walking or cycling to help burn calories.

3. **Increase Duration Gradually**: Start with short sessions and gradually increase the duration as your body becomes more accustomed to the exercises.

4. **Combine with Healthy Eating**: Complement your somatic routine with mindful eating practices. Pay attention to your body's hunger cues and nutritional needs.

Integrating Specific Exercises for Weight Loss

1. **Dynamic Cat-Cow**: Speed up the Cat-Cow stretch slightly to increase your heart rate while maintaining mindfulness.

2. **Active Pelvic Tilts**: Add a small lift of your hips off the ground during pelvic tilts to engage the core muscles more.

3. **Leg Extensions with Resistance**: Use light ankle weights during leg extensions for added resistance.

4. **Mindful Cardio**: Include a session of mindful walking or swimming where you focus on the sensation of movement and breath.

Mindfulness and Emotional Well-Being

1. **Mindful Breathing**: Incorporate breathing exercises to manage stress, as stress can often lead to overeating or unhealthy eating habits.

2. **Meditation for Self-Acceptance**: Practice meditation focusing on self-compassion and acceptance, which is crucial for a healthy weight loss journey.

Monitoring and Adjusting Your Routine

1. **Listen to Your Body**: Pay attention to how your body feels during and after exercises. Adjust the intensity and duration accordingly.

2. **Regularly Assess Your Goals**: As you progress, reassess your goals and modify your routine to align with any new objectives.

3. **Seek Professional Guidance**: If possible, consult with a somatic exercise expert or a physical therapist for personalized advice.

Staying Motivated and Consistent

1. **Set Realistic Expectations**: Understand that weight loss with somatic exercises is a gradual process.

2. **Celebrate Small Achievements**: Acknowledge and celebrate small milestones in your journey.

3. **Create a Support System**: Engage with a community or find a partner who shares similar goals for mutual support and motivation.

Conclusion

Customizing your somatic routine for weight loss involves a blend of mindful, body-awareness exercises with lifestyle changes that promote overall well-being. By focusing on gentle, sustainable movements and combining them with healthy eating and stress management, you can achieve and maintain your weight loss goals in a harmonious and healthy way. Remember, the key is consistency and listening to your body's needs.

Chapter 5: Deepening Your Practice

Advanced Somatic Exercises

As you progress in your somatic practice, incorporating advanced exercises can deepen your body awareness and enhance your physical capabilities. These exercises are more challenging and require a good foundation in basic somatic movements.

1. Rotational Pelvic Clock

Purpose: Enhances pelvic mobility and awareness.

Steps:

1. Lie on your back with knees bent and feet flat on the floor.

2. Imagine a clock on your pelvis; 12 o'clock is your navel, and 6 o'clock is your pubic bone.

3. Slowly tilt your pelvis towards each "hour" of the clock in a smooth, circular motion.

4. Reverse the direction after completing one full circle.

2. Full-Body Scan and Release

Purpose: Promotes full-body awareness and relaxation.

Steps:

1. Lie in a comfortable position and close your eyes.

2. Mentally scan your body from head to toe, noticing any areas of tension.

3. Gently tense and then relax each part of your body, starting from your feet and moving upwards.

4. Focus on the sensation of release in each area.

3. Cross-Lateral Extensions

Purpose: Improves coordination and cross-body awareness.

Steps:

1. Lie on your back with arms extended overhead.

2. Slowly raise your right arm and left leg simultaneously, keeping them straight.

3. Lower them and then raise your left arm and right leg.

4. Continue alternating in a slow, controlled manner.

4. Somatic Squats

Purpose: Builds lower body strength and flexibility.

Steps:

1. Stand with feet hip-width apart.

2. Perform a squat while maintaining deep awareness of your body's movements and sensations.

3. Focus on the fluidity and alignment of your movement rather than depth or speed.

4. Return to standing, observing the sensations in your muscles.

5. Somatic Plank Variations

Purpose: Strengthens the core with mindful engagement.

Steps:

1. Begin in a plank position, with your forearms and toes on the ground.

2. Maintain this position with a focus on the sensations in your core and back.

3. For variation, gently shift your weight from side to side or front to back.

4. Keep your movements slow and controlled.

6. Dynamic Spinal Twists

Purpose: Enhances spinal flexibility and releases tension.

Steps:

1. Sit on the floor with your legs extended.

2. Cross your right foot over your left thigh, placing it flat on the floor.

3. Place your right hand behind you and gently twist to the right, using your left arm for leverage.

4. Hold for a few breaths, focusing on the twisting sensation, then switch sides.

7. Somatic Yoga Poses

Purpose: Integrates somatic awareness into yoga practice.

Steps:

1. Choose yoga poses that challenge your balance and flexibility.

2. Perform each pose with a deep focus on the sensations and alignment in your body.

3. Use breath to deepen the awareness and fluidity of the movements.

Conclusion

Advanced somatic exercises are about deepening the connection between your mind and body. As you practice these exercises, maintain a focus on internal sensations and mindfulness. Remember, the goal is not to push your body but to explore its capabilities with awareness and respect. As always, listen to your body and adjust the exercises to suit your individual needs and limitations.

Integrating Mindfulness with Physical Movement

Combining mindfulness with physical movement creates a holistic exercise experience that benefits both the mind and body. This integration is key in practices like yoga, tai chi, and somatic exercises. Here's how to effectively integrate mindfulness into your physical movements.

1. Setting Intentions

- **Begin with Intent**: Before starting, set a clear intention for your practice. This could be to focus on your breath, to move with grace, or simply to be present.

- **Mindful Preparation**: Spend a few moments in stillness, tuning into your breath and mental state, preparing yourself for mindful movement.

2. Focused Breathing

- **Synchronize Movement with Breath**: In exercises like yoga or tai chi, coordinate your movements with your breathing. For instance, inhale during upward movements and exhale during downward movements.

- **Awareness of Breath**: Keep your focus on the rhythm of your breath, noticing how your body moves in response to each breath.

3. Body Awareness

- **Notice Bodily Sensations**: As you move, pay attention to the sensations in different parts of your body. Feel the muscle stretch, the joint rotation, and any tension or ease.

- **Gentle Adjustments**: Make small, mindful adjustments to your posture and movement to align better and move more efficiently.

4. Mindful Observation

- **Non-Judgmental Awareness**: Observe your abilities and limitations without judgment. Acknowledge your progress and areas for improvement with kindness and patience.

- **Stay Present**: If your mind wanders, gently bring your focus back to your body and breath.

5. Dynamic Movement and Flow

- **Fluidity in Movement**: In exercises like dance or flowing yoga sequences, focus on the flow and transition between movements, creating a sense of fluidity and grace.

- **Energy and Emotion**: Be aware of the energy and emotions that arise during movement. Allow these feelings to express themselves through your physical actions.

6. Ending with Mindfulness

- **Cool Down Mindfully**: Conclude your session with a period of cool-down. Slow your movements and bring your attention back to slower, deeper breaths.

- **Reflective Pause**: End with a moment of stillness, reflecting on your practice, the sensations in your body, and your mental state.

7. Daily Integration

- **Mindful Daily Activities**: Practice mindfulness in everyday movements, such as walking, climbing stairs, or performing household chores. Focus on the movement and your interaction with your environment.

- **Regular Check-ins**: Throughout the day, pause to notice your posture, breathing, and any areas of tension or relaxation in your body.

Conclusion

Integrating mindfulness into physical movement enhances the exercise experience, making it more holistic and beneficial. It allows for a deeper connection with the body, improves focus and mental clarity, and promotes a sense of peace and well-being. This practice is not just about physical fitness but about nurturing a harmonious relationship between the mind and body.

Building a Daily Somatic Routine

Creating a daily somatic routine is an excellent way to maintain consistency in your practice and reap the long-term benefits of somatic exercises. Here's a guide to help you establish a routine that fits into your daily life.

1. Establishing a Routine

- **Set a Specific Time**: Choose a time of day when you can consistently practice, whether it's morning, afternoon, or evening. Consistency is key.

- **Start Small**: Begin with a short duration that feels manageable, like 10-15 minutes, and gradually increase as you become more comfortable.

- **Create a Dedicated Space**: Find a quiet, comfortable space in your home where you can practice without interruptions.

2. Warming Up

- **Gentle Stretching**: Start with some gentle stretches to warm up your muscles and joints. This could include neck rolls, shoulder shrugs, and arm circles.

- **Mindful Breathing**: Spend a few minutes focusing on your breath, using deep diaphragmatic breathing to center yourself.

3. Core Somatic Exercises

- **Pelvic Tilts**: Begin with pelvic tilts to bring awareness to your core and lower back.

- **Cat-Cow Stretch**: Transition to the Cat-Cow stretch, synchronizing your movement with your breath.

- **Rotational Movements**: Include rotational movements like gentle spinal twists to increase spinal mobility.

- **Leg and Arm Movements**: Incorporate slow leg and arm movements to connect with the extremities.

4. Mindfulness Integration

- **Focus on Sensations**: As you move, concentrate on the sensations in your body. Notice how each part feels and how they work together.

- **Breath Awareness**: Continue to focus on your breath, ensuring it remains steady and deep.

5. Advanced Techniques (As Progressed)

- **Incorporate More Challenging Exercises**: As you get comfortable, add more advanced exercises like cross-lateral extensions or dynamic spinal twists.

- **Experiment with Flow**: Try transitioning smoothly from one exercise to another, creating a flow of movement.

6. Cool Down

- **Slow Down Movements**: Gradually slow your movements, allowing your heart rate to return to normal.

- **End with Relaxation**: Conclude with a relaxation exercise, like the constructive rest position, focusing on releasing any remaining tension.

7. Reflection

- **Mindful Meditation**: Spend a few minutes in meditation, reflecting on your practice and its effects on your body and mind.

- **Journaling**: Consider keeping a journal to note your experiences, feelings, and progress.

8. Incorporating Somatics into Daily Life

- **Mindful Daily Activities**: Practice mindfulness and body awareness in everyday activities like walking, sitting, or even doing household chores.

- **Regular Breaks**: Take short breaks throughout your day for quick somatic exercises or deep breathing to maintain body awareness and reduce stress.

Conclusion

Building a daily somatic routine is a personal journey that requires patience and consistency. Tailor your practice to your body's needs and daily schedule. Over time, this routine will not only enhance your physical well-being but also deepen your connection to your body, improving your overall quality of life.

Chapter 6: Nutrition for the Somatic Journey

The Importance of Nutrition in Somatic Wellness
Understanding the Connection

Nutrition plays a crucial role in somatic wellness, a holistic approach that emphasizes the interconnectedness of body and mind. Proper nutrition supports the physical body, which in turn impacts mental and emotional well-being.

Nutritional Foundations for Somatic Health

1. **Balanced Diet**: A diet rich in fruits, vegetables, whole grains, lean proteins, and healthy fats provides the necessary nutrients for bodily function and supports overall health.

2. **Hydration**: Adequate water intake is essential for joint lubrication, muscle function, and overall cellular health.

3. **Mindful Eating**: Practicing mindfulness in eating habits ensures that food intake is aligned with the body's needs and promotes better digestion and satisfaction.

Nutrient Impact on Body Function

- **Energy Levels**: Balanced nutrition ensures steady energy levels, which is crucial for maintaining an active lifestyle and participating in somatic exercises.

- **Muscle and Joint Health**: Proteins, omega-3 fatty acids, and antioxidants help in muscle recovery and joint health, important for movement-based practices.

- **Nervous System Support**: B-vitamins and magnesium are vital for the nervous system, influencing muscle relaxation and stress response.

The Role of Gut Health

- **Gut-Brain Axis**: The gut and brain are directly linked; a healthy gut contributes to a balanced mood and cognitive function, impacting the somatic experience.

- **Probiotics and Prebiotics**: Including foods rich in probiotics and prebiotics can improve gut health, thereby enhancing overall well-being.

Nutrition for Recovery and Healing

- **Post-Exercise Nutrition**: Consuming the right balance of proteins and carbohydrates after somatic exercises aids in muscle recovery and replenishes energy stores.

- **Anti-Inflammatory Foods**: Foods with anti-inflammatory properties can help in reducing muscle soreness and joint pain, which can be beneficial for those engaged in regular somatic practices.

Personalized Nutrition

- **Individual Dietary Needs**: Recognize that each body is different; what works for one may not work for another. Personalize your diet based on your body's responses, health conditions, and goals.

- **Consultation with Professionals**: Consider consulting a nutritionist or dietitian to create a diet plan that aligns with your somatic wellness goals.

- **Pre- and Post-Exercise Meals**: Plan meals around your exercise routine to ensure your body has the fuel it needs for activity and recovery.

- **Mindful Eating Practices**: Incorporate mindfulness into eating as you do with somatic exercises, paying attention to the flavors, textures, and sensations of eating.

Conclusion

In somatic wellness, nutrition is not just about eating healthily; it's about understanding and respecting the body's nutritional needs and how they relate to physical and mental health. A balanced, mindful approach to nutrition can significantly enhance the benefits of somatic practices, leading to a more harmonious and holistic state of well-being.

Nutritional Principles Aligned with Somatic Practices

When aligning nutrition with somatic practices, the focus is on holistic well-being, where diet supports both the physical movements and the overall balance of the mind and body. Here are key nutritional principles that complement somatic wellness:

1. Wholesome and Natural Foods

- **Whole Foods**: Focus on whole, unprocessed foods that are close to their natural state. These include fruits, vegetables, whole grains, nuts, seeds, and lean proteins.

- **Minimizing Processed Foods**: Reduce intake of processed and refined foods, which often contain additives and preservatives that can affect body and mind.

2. Balanced and Varied Diet

- **Macronutrient Balance**: Ensure a good balance of carbohydrates, proteins, and fats to provide energy, support muscle health, and maintain cellular functions.

- **Diverse Nutrients**: Incorporate a variety of foods to ensure a wide range of vitamins, minerals, and antioxidants that support overall health.

3. Mindful Eating

- **Eating with Awareness**: Practice being fully present while eating, paying attention to the taste, texture, and sensations of food.

- **Listening to the Body**: Eat in response to hunger cues and stop when full. This principle aligns with the somatic focus on internal body awareness.

4. Hydration

- **Adequate Water Intake**: Water is essential for joint lubrication, temperature regulation, and overall bodily functions. Ensure you're drinking enough water throughout the day.

- **Limiting Stimulants**: Reduce intake of caffeine and alcohol, which can dehydrate the body and affect mental clarity.

5. Anti-Inflammatory Foods

- **Incorporate Anti-Inflammatory Ingredients**: Foods like turmeric, ginger, berries, green leafy vegetables, and omega-3 rich foods (like salmon and flaxseeds) can help reduce inflammation, aiding in muscle recovery and joint health.

6. Gut Health

- **Probiotics and Prebiotics**: Include foods that promote gut health, such as yogurt, kefir, sauerkraut, and high-fiber fruits and vegetables. A healthy gut is linked to improved mood and cognitive function.

7. Timing of Meals

- **Aligning Meals with Activity**: Time your meals to support your energy needs. For example, a balanced meal a few hours before somatic exercises for energy, and a protein-rich meal afterward for muscle recovery.

8. Personalization

- **Individual Dietary Needs**: Tailor your diet to your personal health needs, preferences, and any specific goals or medical conditions.

- **Regular Adjustments**: Be open to adjusting your diet as your somatic practice evolves or as your body's needs change.

Conclusion

Nutrition in somatic practices is not just about what you eat, but also how and when you eat. It's about creating harmony between your diet and your physical and mental states. By adopting these principles, you can support your somatic journey, enhancing both your physical movements and your overall sense of well-being.

Meal Planning and Healthy Eating Habits

Adopting healthy eating habits and effective meal planning can significantly contribute to overall well-being. These practices are essential for maintaining energy levels, improving body function, and supporting somatic practices.

1. Start with a Plan

- **Assess Nutritional Needs**: Based on your activity level, health goals, and any dietary restrictions.

- **Plan Your Meals in Advance**: This helps to avoid last-minute unhealthy choices. Plan for a week in advance, including all meals and snacks.

- **Grocery List and Shopping**: Make a list based on your meal plan to ensure you buy only what you need, focusing on fresh, whole ingredients.

2. Balanced Meals

- **Include a Variety of Foods**: Each meal should have a balance of carbohydrates (preferably complex carbs like whole grains), proteins, and healthy fats.

- **Colorful Vegetables and Fruits**: Aim for a variety of colors in your diet, as different colors represent different nutrients and antioxidants.

3. Mindful Eating Practices

- **Eat Without Distractions**: Avoid eating while working, watching TV, or using your phone. Mindful eating helps in better digestion and portion control.

- **Chew Thoroughly**: Take time to chew your food properly. This aids in digestion and can increase the feeling of fullness.

4. Hydration

- **Drink Plenty of Water**: Carry a water bottle and sip throughout the day, not just during meals.

- **Limit Sugary Drinks**: Reduce the intake of sugary beverages and opt for water, herbal teas, or infused water for hydration.

5. Regular Eating Schedule

- **Consistent Meal Times**: Try to eat at roughly the same times every day. This can regulate your body's hunger signals and improve metabolism.

- **Avoid Late-Night Eating**: Try to have your last meal a few hours before bedtime to ensure proper digestion.

6. Portion Control

- **Use Smaller Plates**: This can help in controlling portion sizes.

- **Listen to Your Body**: Eat until you're comfortably full, not stuffed.

7. Healthy Snacking

- **Plan Healthy Snacks**: Choose snacks like nuts, fruits, yogurt, or whole-grain crackers to keep you energized between meals.

- **Avoid Processed Snacks**: Steer clear of snacks high in sugar, salt, and unhealthy fats.

8. Cooking Methods

- **Healthier Cooking Techniques**: Opt for baking, steaming, grilling, or stir-frying instead of deep-frying or sautéing in excessive oil.

- **Experiment with Herbs and Spices**: They add flavor without extra calories and can have additional health benefits.

9. Dealing with Cravings

- **Healthy Alternatives**: Find healthy alternatives to satisfy cravings, like dark chocolate instead of milk chocolate, or baked sweet potato fries instead of regular fries.

- **Understand and Manage Cravings**: Sometimes, cravings can be due to stress, dehydration, or lack of nutrients. Understanding the cause can help manage them effectively.

Conclusion

Meal planning and healthy eating habits are about creating a sustainable and enjoyable approach to food. These practices not only support your physical health but also enhance your somatic experiences by nourishing your body in alignment with its needs. Remember, the goal is to develop a positive relationship with food, where it becomes a source of nourishment and pleasure.

Chapter 7: Guided Audio Meditations

Purpose and Benefits of Audio Meditations

Understanding Audio Meditations

Audio meditations are guided experiences where an instructor leads you through a meditation practice, often accompanied by soothing background music or natural sounds. These meditations are accessible via recordings, apps, or online platforms.

Purpose of Audio Meditations

1. **Guidance for Beginners**: They provide structure and guidance for those new to meditation, making it easier to engage in the practice.

2. **Focus Assistance**: The audio guidance helps keep the mind focused, which can be challenging for many during silent meditation.

3. **Variety and Flexibility**: Offers a variety of meditation styles and lengths, catering to different preferences and schedules.

Benefits of Audio Meditations

1. **Stress Reduction**: Regular meditation has been shown to reduce stress and its physical and psychological effects.

2. **Enhanced Concentration**: Improves focus and attention, which can benefit all areas of life, including work and personal relationships.

3. **Emotional Balance**: Helps in managing emotions, leading to greater emotional stability and resilience.

4. **Improved Sleep**: Certain audio meditations are designed to promote relaxation and can be an effective tool for combating insomnia and improving sleep quality.

5. **Increased Self-Awareness**: Fosters a deeper understanding of oneself and can lead to increased mindfulness in daily life.

6. **Accessibility**: Audio meditations make the practice accessible to a wider audience, including those who may not have access to in-person guidance.

7. **Customizable Experience**: Listeners can choose meditations based on their current needs, whether it's a quick relaxation session, a sleep aid, or a deeper exploration of mindfulness.

8. **Enhanced Relaxation**: The combination of guided instructions and soothing sounds can quickly induce a state of relaxation.

Integration with Somatic Practices

- **Pre-Exercise Centering**: Listening to a short meditation before engaging in somatic exercises can help center the mind and prepare the body.

- **Post-Exercise Reflection**: A calming meditation after physical activity can enhance the integration of the mind-body benefits experienced during the exercise.

Conclusion

Audio meditations are a valuable tool for enhancing mental clarity, emotional stability, and overall well-being. They complement somatic practices by deepening the mind-body connection and making meditation a more accessible and varied practice. Whether you are a beginner or an experienced practitioner, incorporating audio meditations into your routine can offer profound benefits.

How to Use Guided Meditations Alongside Somatic Exercises

Integrating guided meditations with somatic exercises can create a comprehensive mind-body wellness routine. Here's a step-by-step approach to effectively combine these practices.

1. Setting the Environment

- **Create a Calm Space**: Choose a quiet, comfortable area for both your meditation and somatic exercises. Ensure the space is free from distractions.

- **Gather Necessary Materials**: Have a mat, comfortable clothing, and any meditation aids (like headphones or speakers) ready.

2. Starting with Meditation

- **Begin with a Short Meditation**: Start your routine with a 5-10 minute guided meditation to center your mind and bring focus to your body. This can help in cultivating mindfulness, which enhances the effectiveness of somatic exercises.

- **Focus on Breath**: Use the meditation to bring awareness to your breathing, establishing a rhythm that you can maintain throughout your somatic practice.

3. Transitioning to Somatic Exercises

- **Gradual Transition**: After the meditation, slowly transition to your somatic exercises. Maintain the mindful state cultivated during meditation.

- **Incorporate Mindful Movement**: As you move through somatic exercises, remain fully present and attentive to the sensations in your body, your alignment, and the quality of your movements.

4. During Somatic Exercises

- **Use the Breath as an Anchor**: Keep your breathing steady and synchronized with your movements. This not only aids in physical execution but also keeps you anchored in the present moment.

- **Body Awareness**: Pay close attention to how your body feels with each movement. Notice any areas of tension, ease, or particular sensitivity.

5. Closing with Meditation

- **End with a Meditation**: Conclude your routine with another guided meditation. This could be a relaxation or gratitude meditation to assimilate the benefits of the somatic exercises.

- **Reflect on the Experience**: Use this time to reflect on how your body and mind feel post-exercise. Observe any changes in your mental or physical state.

6. Regular Practice

- **Consistency is Key**: Incorporate this combined practice of meditation and somatic exercises into your regular routine for maximum benefit.

- **Vary Your Practices**: Experiment with different types of meditations and somatic exercises to keep the routine engaging and cover various aspects of mind-body wellness.

7. Integrating Throughout the Day

- **Mindful Moments**: Besides your dedicated practice time, find moments throughout the day for brief periods of mindfulness or gentle somatic movements, especially during times of stress or prolonged sitting.

8. Listening to Your Body

- **Adapt as Needed**: Be responsive to your body's needs. Some days you might focus more on meditation, while on others, you may engage more deeply in somatic movements.

Conclusion

Combining guided meditations with somatic exercises offers a holistic approach to wellness, addressing both mental and physical health. This integrated practice can improve focus, reduce stress, enhance body awareness, and contribute to overall well-being. By practicing regularly, you can deepen your mind-body connection and experience a more balanced and harmonious state of being.

Chapter 8: Somatic Wellness in Everyday Life

Incorporating Somatic Practices into Daily Routines

Integrating somatic practices into your daily life can significantly enhance your overall well-being. These practices help in developing a deeper awareness of your body and its connection to your mental state. Here's how to seamlessly incorporate them into your everyday routine.

1. Morning Ritual

- **Gentle Wake-up Stretch**: Begin your day with simple stretches or a few minutes of mindful movement to awaken the body.

- **Breathing Exercises**: Practice deep breathing or a short guided breathing meditation to center yourself for the day.

2. Integrating with Work or Study

- **Mindful Breaks**: Take short breaks throughout the day to practice somatic exercises like neck rolls, shoulder shrugs, or pelvic tilts.

- **Conscious Posture**: Be aware of your posture while sitting or standing. Adjust regularly to reduce tension and maintain alignment.

3. Mindful Movement Breaks

- **Walk Mindfully**: During walks, focus on the sensation of your feet touching the ground, your breathing, and the movements of your body.

- **Stretching Sessions**: Incorporate stretching or gentle yoga poses during breaks to release physical tension.

4. Mindful Eating

- **Somatic Awareness While Eating**: Pay attention to the tastes, textures, and sensations while eating. Chew slowly and savor each bite.

- **Listening to Hunger Cues**: Use somatic principles to tune into your body's hunger signals and eat accordingly.

5. Evening Wind-down

- **Relaxation Exercises**: Practice relaxing somatic exercises in the evening to unwind. This could include gentle stretching or body scans.

- **Guided Meditation**: End your day with a guided meditation to relax your mind and prepare for restful sleep.

6. Physical Activity Integration

- **Somatic Elements in Exercise**: Incorporate somatic principles into your regular exercise routine, focusing on body awareness and mindful movement.

- **Outdoor Activities**: Engage in outdoor activities like hiking or cycling with a focus on the sensory experience.

7. Stress Management

- **Mindful Response to Stress**: When feeling stressed, take a moment to practice deep breathing or a quick somatic exercise to center yourself.

- **Emotional Awareness**: Use somatic techniques to become more aware of how emotions manifest in your body and address them mindfully.

8. Household Activities

- **Somatic Awareness in Chores**: Be mindful of your body and movements while doing household chores. Use these activities as an opportunity to practice good posture and body mechanics.

9. Regular Reflection

- **Reflect on Your Practices**: At the end of each day, reflect on how somatic practices have influenced your body and mind. Note any changes in your stress levels, body awareness, and overall well-being.

Conclusion

Incorporating somatic practices into your daily routines can lead to greater bodily awareness, reduced stress, and improved overall health. These practices encourage a more mindful, connected approach to daily activities, enhancing both mental and physical wellness.

Overcoming Common Challenges and Staying Motivated

Adopting and maintaining a regular somatic practice can be challenging. Here are strategies to overcome common obstacles and stay motivated.

1. Lack of Time

- **Integrate into Daily Activities**: Find ways to incorporate somatic exercises into your daily routine, like doing pelvic tilts while at your desk or mindful breathing during your commute.

- **Short Sessions**: Remember that even short sessions are beneficial. If you can't commit to a long practice, a few minutes can still make a difference.

2. Difficulty Staying Consistent

- **Set a Schedule**: Create a regular schedule for your practice. Consistency is key to forming a habit.

- **Reminders and Alarms**: Use reminders or alarms on your phone or in your companion app to prompt your practice.

3. Boredom or Lack of Engagement

- **Vary Your Routine**: Change your somatic exercises regularly to keep the practice fresh and engaging.

- **Explore New Techniques**: Try different somatic disciplines or incorporate new mindfulness activities to maintain interest.

4. Physical Limitations or Discomfort

- **Listen to Your Body**: Adjust exercises to accommodate any physical limitations or pain. Somatic practices should be gentle and not cause discomfort.

- **Consult a Professional**: If needed, seek advice from a somatic practitioner, physical therapist, or healthcare provider.

5. Slow Progress or Lack of Visible Results

- **Set Realistic Expectations**: Understand that progress in somatic practices is often subtle and gradual.

- **Focus on Non-Physical Benefits**: Recognize and value the mental and emotional benefits of your practice, like reduced stress or improved mood.

6. Waning Motivation

- **Remember Your Goals**: Revisit the reasons why you started somatic practices. Reminding yourself of your goals can reignite motivation.

- **Track Your Progress**: Use the companion app to track your progress and see how far you've come.

7. Isolation in Practice

- **Join a Community**: Engage with online forums or local groups practicing somatics. Sharing experiences and tips can be motivating.

- **Practice with Friends or Family**: Having a practice partner can increase accountability and make the experience more enjoyable.

8. Integrating Mindfulness

- **Mindful Reflection**: After each session, spend a few minutes reflecting on how your body and mind feel. This can deepen your connection to the practice.

- **Mindfulness Throughout the Day**: Practice mindfulness in everyday activities to reinforce the principles of somatic wellness.

Conclusion

Overcoming challenges in somatic practices often involves a combination of strategic planning, mindset shifts, and community support. By addressing these common obstacles, you can maintain a consistent and fulfilling somatic practice, leading to enhanced physical and mental well-being.

Long-term Benefits of Somatic Wellness

Somatic wellness, which emphasizes a holistic approach to physical health by integrating the mind and body, offers a range of long-term benefits. These benefits extend beyond immediate physical improvements, contributing to overall life quality and well-being.

1. Improved Body Awareness

- **Enhanced Sensory Perception**: Regular somatic practice increases your awareness of bodily sensations, leading to a deeper understanding of your body's needs and responses.

- **Prevention of Injury**: This heightened body awareness can help in preventing injuries by recognizing and addressing minor issues before they become major.

2. Stress Reduction and Emotional Regulation

- **Reduced Stress Levels**: Somatic practices, especially those incorporating mindfulness and deep breathing, are effective in reducing stress.

- **Better Emotional Balance**: These practices can lead to improved emotional regulation, helping you to manage anxiety and depression more effectively.

3. Increased Flexibility and Mobility

- **Greater Flexibility**: Somatic exercises often lead to improved flexibility, as they gently stretch and strengthen the body.

- **Enhanced Mobility**: Over time, these practices can enhance your range of motion and mobility, making daily activities easier and more enjoyable.

4. Improved Posture and Alignment

- **Better Posture**: Somatic practices foster an awareness of alignment and posture, leading to natural improvements in how you stand, sit, and move.

- **Reduced Pain**: Improved posture can alleviate pain, especially in areas like the back and neck, often affected by poor posture.

5. Enhanced Mental Clarity and Focus

- **Increased Mental Focus**: The mindfulness aspect of somatic practices can sharpen your concentration and mental clarity.

- **Cognitive Benefits**: Regular practice can lead to enhanced cognitive function, including better memory and problem-solving skills.

6. Strengthening and Toning of Muscles

- **Muscle Toning**: Somatic exercises engage various muscle groups, leading to a more toned and balanced physique.

- **Functional Strength**: These practices develop functional strength, which is crucial for daily activities and overall physical resilience.

7. Improved Sleep Quality

- **Relaxation and Sleep**: The relaxation techniques inherent in somatic practices can lead to improved sleep quality, aiding in recovery and rejuvenation.

- **Reduced Insomnia Symptoms**: Regular practice can also help in managing insomnia and other sleep disturbances.

8. Enhanced Overall Well-being

- **Holistic Health Improvement**: Somatic wellness encourages a comprehensive approach to health, considering physical, mental, and emotional aspects.

- **Quality of Life**: By promoting harmony between the mind and body, somatic practices can significantly improve your overall quality of life.

9. Healthy Aging

- **Age Gracefully**: Somatic practices support healthy aging, maintaining flexibility, strength, and mental acuity as you grow older.

- **Prevention of Age-Related Issues**: These practices can help in preventing or managing age-related health issues, such as arthritis and osteoporosis.

Conclusion

The long-term benefits of somatic wellness practices are profound and multifaceted. They contribute not only to physical health but also to emotional balance, mental clarity, and overall life satisfaction. By regularly engaging in these practices, you can enjoy a more harmonious, healthy, and fulfilling life.

Chapter 9: Beyond the Book - Continuing Your Journey

Additional Resources and Continuing Education for Somatic Wellness

To deepen your understanding and practice of somatic wellness, it's beneficial to engage with a variety of resources and opportunities for continuing education. Here are some valuable resources and suggestions:

1. Books and Publications

- **Somatic Wellness Literature**: Read books specifically about somatic exercises, mindfulness, and body awareness. Look for works by pioneers in the field like Thomas Hanna or Moshe Feldenkrais.

- **Research Journals**: Subscribe to journals or online publications that focus on holistic health, mind-body integration, and somatic practices.

2. Online Courses and Workshops

- **Digital Learning Platforms**: Enroll in online courses on platforms like Udemy, Coursera, or Mindvalley that offer programs in mindfulness, meditation, and somatic therapy.

- **Workshops and Webinars**: Attend workshops or webinars hosted by experts in somatic wellness. These can often be found through wellness centers or professional networks.

3. Professional Training and Certifications

- **Certification Programs**: If you are interested in teaching or deepening your practice, consider enrolling in certification programs for somatic therapy, yoga, or Pilates.

- **Continuing Education Credits**: For professionals, look for courses that offer continuing education credits in related fields.

4. Networking and Professional Groups

- **Join Professional Associations**: Become a member of professional groups or associations related to somatic practices, holistic health, or wellness coaching.

- **Networking Events**: Attend conferences, seminars, and networking events to connect with peers and learn about the latest trends and research.

5. Community Classes and Groups

- **Local Wellness Groups**: Participate in community classes or meetups focusing on somatic exercises, yoga, tai chi, or dance.

- **Practice Groups**: Join or form practice groups to share experiences and techniques in somatic wellness.

6. Retreats and Immersive Experiences

- **Wellness Retreats**: Attend retreats that focus on somatic practices and holistic wellness. These can provide immersive experiences for deeper learning and practice.

- **Mindfulness and Meditation Retreats**: These retreats can deepen your mindfulness practice, an integral part of somatic wellness.

7. Podcasts and Videos

- **Educational Podcasts**: Listen to podcasts that explore topics on mindfulness, somatic therapy, and holistic health.

- **Instructional Videos**: Use platforms like YouTube for instructional videos on somatic exercises and techniques.

8. Apps and Technology

- **Wellness and Meditation Apps**: Utilize apps that offer guided meditations, mindfulness exercises, and educational content on somatic practices.

- **Virtual Reality (VR) Experiences**: Explore VR platforms that offer immersive wellness and mindfulness experiences.

9. Personal Research and Self-Study

- **Stay Informed**: Regularly read articles, blogs, and studies about somatic wellness to stay up-to-date with the latest information.

- **Personal Experimentation**: Apply what you learn in your practice, experimenting with different techniques and approaches.

Conclusion

The journey of somatic wellness is ongoing, and engaging with these resources can provide valuable knowledge, skills, and inspiration. Whether you're looking to deepen your personal practice or pursue professional opportunities in the field, these resources offer a wealth of information and experiences to support your growth and development in somatic wellness.

Joining the Somatic Wellness Community

Becoming part of a somatic wellness community can significantly enrich your practice and understanding of somatic principles. Here's how to connect with and become an active member of this community.

1. Local Classes and Groups

- **Participate in Local Workshops**: Look for yoga studios, wellness centers, or community centers that offer classes in somatic practices such as Feldenkrais, Alexander Technique, or body-mind centering.

- **Community Meetups**: Join local meetups or groups focused on mindfulness and body awareness practices. These can often be found on social platforms like Meetup.com.

2. Online Forums and Social Media

- **Engage in Online Communities**: Become active in online forums or social media groups dedicated to somatic wellness. This is a great way to connect with a global community.

- **Follow Influencers and Experts**: Follow somatic wellness practitioners and experts on platforms like

Instagram, YouTube, or Twitter to stay updated on new insights and practices.

3. Networking Events and Conferences

- **Attend Conferences and Seminars**: Look for conferences, seminars, or symposiums that focus on somatic practices. These events are opportunities for learning and networking.

- **Professional Associations**: Joining professional associations related to somatic practices can provide access to exclusive events and resources.

4. Collaborative Learning

- **Study Groups**: Form or join study groups with peers to discuss and explore somatic concepts and practices.

- **Interactive Workshops**: Participate in interactive workshops where you can practice somatic exercises and share experiences with others.

5. Volunteering and Community Service

- **Volunteer Opportunities**: Engage in volunteer work related to wellness and somatic practices. Teaching somatic exercises in community centers or schools can be rewarding.

- **Community Projects**: Collaborate in community projects or initiatives that promote holistic wellness and somatic practices.

6. Retreats and Immersive Experiences

- **Join Wellness Retreats**: Attend retreats that focus on somatic wellness. These can offer immersive experiences and the opportunity to connect deeply with others who share similar interests.

- **Travel and Learn**: Consider traveling to places known for their emphasis on holistic wellness and somatic practices for a more immersive experience.

7. Creating Content and Sharing Experiences

- **Start a Blog or Vlog**: Share your somatic journey through blogging or vlogging. This not only helps others learn from your experiences but also establishes you within the community.

- **Host Webinars or Podcasts**: Hosting online sessions on topics related to somatic wellness can attract like-minded individuals and facilitate community building.

8. Continuous Learning and Sharing

- **Regularly Share Learnings**: Share what you learn from courses, books, or personal experiences with the community.

- **Mentorship**: As you gain more experience, consider mentoring newcomers to the somatic wellness community.

Conclusion

Joining and contributing to the somatic wellness community can be a fulfilling and enriching experience. It offers opportunities for personal growth, learning, networking, and sharing in a collective journey towards holistic health and well-being. By actively engaging with these various platforms and opportunities, you can deepen your connection to the somatic wellness world and contribute to its growth and diversity.

Next Steps in Your Somatic Wellness Journey

Embarking on a journey of somatic wellness is a lifelong process of learning, growing, and deepening your understanding of the mind-body connection. Here are steps to further this journey, ensuring continuous development and enrichment.

1. Deepen Your Practice

- **Expand Your Knowledge**: Continuously seek out new information about somatic practices through books, courses, and workshops.

- **Experiment with Different Techniques**: Try various somatic methods like Feldenkrais, Alexander Technique, or yoga to see what resonates with you and your body.

2. Integrate Somatic Principles into Daily Life

- **Daily Mind-Body Check-ins**: Make it a habit to check in with your body and mind throughout the day, practicing mindfulness and body awareness.

- **Apply Somatic Concepts in Activities**: Use principles of somatic wellness in everyday activities, such as mindful walking, conscious breathing, or ergonomics in your workspace.

3. Join a Community

- **Participate in Somatic Wellness Groups**: Join local or online communities to share experiences and gain support.

- **Attend Retreats and Workshops**: These can provide immersive experiences and the opportunity to learn from experts.

4. Monitor and Reflect on Your Progress

- **Use a Journal**: Keep a journal to track your progress, reflect on your experiences, and note any changes in your body and mind.

- **Set Regular Goals**: Continuously set and review goals related to your somatic practice to keep your journey focused and purposeful.

5. Share Your Experience

- **Teach or Mentor Others**: Share your knowledge and experiences with others interested in somatic wellness. Teaching can be a powerful way to deepen your own understanding.

- **Create Content**: If you're inclined, start a blog, podcast, or social media account to discuss and share your journey and insights.

6. Maintain Balance

- **Holistic Approach to Wellness**: Ensure that your somatic practice is part of a balanced approach to wellness that includes nutrition, mental health, and other forms of exercise.

- **Regularly Assess Balance**: Periodically assess how well your somatic practice is integrated with other aspects of your life and health.

7. Explore Professional Development

- **Certification Programs**: If deeply passionate, consider becoming certified in a somatic practice to professionalize your passion.

- **Continuing Education**: Engage in continuing education opportunities to stay current with the latest developments in somatic health.

8. Stay Open and Curious

- **Embrace Change and Growth**: Be open to how your practice and understanding might evolve. Stay curious and willing to adapt your approach.

- **Seek New Experiences**: Continually seek new experiences and challenges within the realm of somatic wellness to further your growth.

Conclusion

Your somatic wellness journey is uniquely yours. It's about finding what works for you, adapting it to your lifestyle, and continuously growing and learning. By staying committed, curious, and engaged, you can make somatic wellness a rewarding and integral part of your life.

Appendices

Glossary of Somatic Terms

In the realm of somatic wellness, certain terms are frequently used to describe concepts and practices. Understanding these terms can deepen your appreciation and practice of somatic exercises. Here's a glossary of key somatic terms:

1. **Somatics**: A field within bodywork and movement studies focusing on the body from the first-person perspective. It involves the perception and experience of one's own body.

2. **Body Awareness**: The conscious knowledge of one's own body parts and movements, often enhanced through somatic practices.

3. **Mindfulness**: The practice of maintaining a nonjudgmental state of heightened or complete awareness of one's thoughts, emotions, or experiences on a moment-to-moment basis.

4. **Kinesthetic Awareness**: The ability to understand and feel the position and movement of the body in space, without relying on sight.

5. **Neuroplasticity**: The ability of the brain to form and reorganize synaptic connections, especially in response to learning or experience or following injury.

6. **Feldenkrais Method**: A somatic educational system designed by Moshé Feldenkrais. It aims to reduce pain

or limitations in movement, to improve physical function, and to promote general well-being.

7. **Alexander Technique**: A process taught to reeducate mind and body into learning new and more efficient ways of moving and breathing, to improve posture and movement, and to relieve chronic stiffness, tension, and stress.

8. **Proprioception**: The sense through which we perceive the position and movement of our body, including the sense of equilibrium.

9. **Diaphragmatic Breathing**: A type of deep breathing that fully engages the diaphragm and is often used in meditation and somatic practices for relaxation.

10. **Constructive Rest Position**: A somatic exercise that involves lying on the back with knees bent and feet flat, used to release tension and align the body.

11. **Body Scan Meditation**: A mindfulness practice that involves mentally scanning the body for areas of tension and relaxation.

12. **Embodiment**: The practice of being in touch with and aware of the body, often used in somatics to describe a deep sense of connection with one's physical self.

Understanding these terms provides a solid foundation for exploring and engaging in somatic wellness practices. They are key to navigating the teachings and literature in this field.

Frequently Asked Questions

What is Somatic Wellness?

Somatic Wellness refers to a holistic approach to health that emphasizes the interconnectedness of the mind and body. It involves practices that focus on internal physical perception and experience, aiming to improve physical function, reduce pain, and enhance overall well-being.

How Does Somatic Practice Differ from Regular Exercise?

While regular exercise often focuses on improving physical fitness, strength, or endurance, somatic practices emphasize internal awareness and the experience of movement. Somatic exercises are typically gentler and more focused on how the body feels during movement, rather than on the intensity or calorie burn.

Can Somatic Practices Help with Stress?

Yes, somatic practices are highly effective in managing stress. They combine physical movement with mindfulness, which helps in reducing mental stress and its physical manifestations like muscle tension.

How Often Should I Practice Somatic Exercises?

The frequency of somatic practice can vary based on individual needs and goals. However, incorporating some form of somatic exercise into your daily routine, even if only for a few minutes, can be beneficial.

Do I Need Special Equipment for Somatic Exercises?

Most somatic exercises do not require special equipment. They can be practiced on a yoga mat or even a comfortable floor space. The key focus is on your body and its movements, rather than external tools.

Are Somatic Practices Suitable for Everyone?

Yes, somatic practices are generally suitable for people of all ages and fitness levels. They are particularly beneficial for those looking for a gentle form of exercise that also promotes mental well-being. However, if you have specific health concerns, it's always best to consult with a healthcare provider before starting any new exercise regimen.

Can Somatic Wellness Improve Mental Health?

Somatic wellness practices have a positive impact on mental health. They promote mindfulness, reduce stress, and can help in managing symptoms of anxiety and depression.

How Can I Incorporate Somatic Practices into My Daily Life?

You can incorporate somatic practices into your daily life by starting your day with mindful breathing or gentle stretching, taking short breaks during the day for body awareness exercises, and ending your day with a relaxation technique like a body scan meditation.

Where Can I Learn Somatic Exercises?

Somatic exercises can be learned from a variety of sources including books, online courses, workshops, and classes offered at yoga studios or wellness centers. It's also possible to find instructional videos and guided sessions online.

Additional Resources and References

Expanding your knowledge and practice in somatic wellness can be greatly enhanced by accessing various resources. Here is a list of additional resources and references that can provide deeper insights and practical guidance:

Books and Literature

1. **"Somatics" by Thomas Hanna**: A foundational book that introduces the concept of somatics and its application in improving physical and mental health.

2. **"The Body Keeps the Score" by Bessel van der Kolk**: Explores the impact of trauma on the body and mind, and discusses somatic practices as a means for healing.

3. **"Awareness Through Movement" by Moshe Feldenkrais**: A guide to the Feldenkrais Method, offering insights into improving function and range of motion through awareness.

4. **"Body Awareness as Healing Therapy: The Case of Nora" by Moshe Feldenkrais**: An illustrative case study demonstrating the transformative power of somatic education.

5. **"Yoga and Somatics for Pain Relief" by Lisa Petersen**: Combines yoga and somatic exercises for pain management and relief.

Online Courses and Educational Platforms

1. **Udemy and Coursera**: Offer various courses on mindfulness, body awareness, and somatic practices.

2. **The Feldenkrais Guild of North America**: Provides online resources and courses on the Feldenkrais Method.

Websites and Online Resources

1. **Somatic Movement Center**: Offers information, articles, and resources on somatic exercises and their benefits.

2. **Mindful.org**: A comprehensive resource for mindfulness and meditation practices, including somatic mindfulness.

Workshops and Retreats

1. **Local Yoga Studios and Wellness Centers**: Often host workshops and classes focusing on somatic practices.

2. **Wellness Retreats**: Offer immersive experiences in somatic wellness, combining practices like yoga, meditation, and bodywork.

Podcasts and Video Channels

1. **The Somatic Podcast**: Explores different aspects of somatics, featuring experts in the field.

2. **YouTube Channels**: Numerous channels provide instructional videos on somatic exercises and mindfulness practices.

Professional Associations and Networks

1. **The International Somatic Movement Education and Therapy Association (ISMETA)**: A professional network offering resources, conferences, and certification information.

2. **The Alexander Technique International**: Provides resources and information about the Alexander Technique, including a directory of practitioners.

Journals and Scientific Publications

1. **Journal of Bodywork and Movement Therapies**: Offers research and articles on various somatic practices and their effects.

2. **International Journal of Yoga Therapy**: Provides insights into therapeutic applications of yoga, often incorporating somatic principles.

Printed in Great Britain
by Amazon

36114329R00059